FORWARD

Before we get started, I would like to let you know what you can find in this guide. First of all, I am not a doctor. I am a Hashimoto's Thyroiditis survivor. I have lived with this auto-immune disease for 10+ years. My experience, including my personal research and findings, can be found here. This guide is not full of the technical terms and explanations as to what Hashimoto's Thyroiditis is. That can easily be found on the internet. I do have some good references to books, doctors, etc., in this guide that can point you in the right direction if you would like more of that.

Quite simply, my goal for this guide is to HELP you get better faster; saving you money, resources and frustration along the way. I hope you will find this useful and ultimately spread the word to family and friends that are affected too. No one should live feeling miserable, with a sense of defeat and no hope for recovery. You can and will feel better after using the information I put together for you here. (Remember, always discuss new supplements, diets and exercise plans with your doctor before trying them). Furthermore, best of luck, and remember, you are not alone.

CONTENTS

INTRODUCTION

Yay! I'm glad you're here and I'm so happy for you! You've just decided to take the next BIG step towards regaining your life back or helping a loved one or a friend feel great and live a happy, Hashimoto's symptom free life. I've been there, and I know, living with Hashimoto's is the worst. You feel miserable. Once you've gotten one symptom under control, another one comes at you and you're left guessing, is this because of my Hashimoto's, or is it something else?

Having Hashimoto's absolutely changed my life and the lives of those living around me. At one point, I felt so sick that I literally thought I was dying. I couldn't think right, my speech was impaired and I was falling asleep at 6 o'clock in the evening. No joke, I thought I had brain cancer. When the phone call came in from the doctor's office, my TSH (mIU/L) was 15 and my TPO antibodies (IU/mL) were 953. Wow! So, I wasn't dying, but I was sick and I needed to get better.

That was January of 2008. Yes, that's right. I've spent the better part of 10+ years seeing doctor after doctor, trying different medications and supplements, taking 100+ blood tests and spending LOTS of money to get to where I am today. The good thing is, I don't want you or any other person to have to endure that. My research and information is here for you, but skipping directly to the Medication and Supplement section without reading the Lab Tests, Results, and Diagnosis section first, won't necessarily help you. You see, everyone who has Hashimoto's is different and their symptoms are different. So let's start at the beginning and work our way to the end. This way you'll know you're asking your doctor the right questions and doing what's best for you.

One last thing. All of the supplements, medications and/or doctors mentioned in this guide do not provide me with compensation for listing them. This is true research and results - period.

LAB TESTS, RESULTS AND DIAGNOSIS

Did you know you could have Hashimoto's and have a normal thyroid test or TSH level? Absolutely! In fact, I'll bet there are thousands more out there walking around right now feeling miserable due to Hashimoto's and don't even know it. The problem is most doctors see a normal thyroid test and tell you it's not your thyroid. They tell you your symptoms are due to something else. Most doctors don't know to check for Thyroid Peroxidase Antibodies. You see, you can have elevated antibodies in your body slowly hindering your thyroid and it can take years (if ever) before your thyroid or TSH levels come back abnormal.

So, the first step I suggest for everyone is to find a functional medicine doctor and/or an integrative medicine doctor. Keep in mind that not all are covered under insurance, so keep looking and checking until you find one. You may have to pay out of pocket and/or drive a little farther to get to one, but it's worth it. Trust me. I have friends that travel across states to see their "special" doctors because they know how much they've helped them. This past year I have been extremely lucky to have found Dr. James Lewerenz from the Longevity Health Institute and Lewerenz Medical Center right here in the metro Detroit, Michigan area. (He does see patients across the country). Before moving to Michigan, I used to see Dr. Oberg in Crystal Lake, Illinois. Point is, you CAN find the right doctor who is willing and able to help you. Now, it is possible you already have a great doctor you trust, who will perform the blood tests you ask for and prescribe the medication you feel is right for you. If so, I encourage you to continue using them. My experience has been that functional and/or integrative medicine doctors tend to approach each individual differently and do what's best for the patient until YOU feel better. They don't just throw conventional medical practices at you and tell you you're fine.

Ok, so by now you've done your research and you've found (or already had) a doctor that can help you. You've made an appointment and now you're ready to get some answers. I don't blame you, but I don't want you to go into the appointment unprepared. Aside from introductions and going over your symptoms (or perhaps you've already been diagnosed with Hashimoto's but still feel horrible), here's a list of the EXACT blood tests you should make sure are ordered for you:

1. Thyroid Peroxidase Antibodies (TPO Antibodies)

2. TSH

3. T4, Free

4. T3, Free

5. T3 Total

6. T3 Reverse

7. Thyroglobulin Antibodies

8. Vitamin D (25-OH Total)

9. Ferritin

10. Comprehensive mineral panel

11. Vitamin B12

12. EBV VCA-IGG

13. EBV VCA-IGM

14. Herpes 1 IGG

15. Herpes 2 IGG

Most functional medicine doctors will also run hormonal testing (Cortisol, DHEA-Sulfate, Estradiol, Estrone, Progesterone, Testosterone, Free Testosterone and Sex Hormone Binding). You might also be asked to do a saliva test to determine if your adrenals are working properly. The saliva test is typically not covered by insurance, and can cost anywhere from $125-$175. So if this is not something you can do, ask your doctor to run a blood test for Alkaline Phosphatase. A low in-range and/or low out-of-range result can indicate Adrenal Fatigue. If your doctor does not run these hormonal tests, no worries. You can always ask to have these run at a later date. It really depends on your insurance and how much it is going to cost you. I would start with tests 1-15 listed above, and in time you can add on the hormonal testing. For purposes of this guide, we'll focus primarily on tests 1-15.

The first seven tests are thyroid related. The

presence of Thyroid Peroxidase Antibodies and/ or Thyroglobulin Antibodies will indicate that you have a Thyroid Disease (or autoimmune disorder) like Hashimoto's or Graves. TSH is Thyroid Stimulating Hormone. This hormone is released by your pituitary gland and it signals your thyroid to release thyroid hormones into your blood stream. If you have a HIGH TSH you have an under active (hypo) thyroid. If you have a LOW TSH you have an over active (hyper) thyroid. T4 is thyroxine. This is produced by your thyroid and is important for growth and metabolism. T3 is triiodothyronine. This is also produced by your thyroid and together with T4 regulates your body temperature, heart rate and metabolism.

The next four tests are vitamins and minerals. If you are feeling tired, slow, mentally foggy, exhausted, etc., it is a good idea to get these tested too. With autoimmunity, there is a direct correlation between low Vitamin D, Vitamin B, Zinc, Magnesium, Calcium, Manganese, Copper and Ferritin (Iron). All of these must be at good levels to help you feel your best. These vitamins and minerals work as anti-inflammatory agents and antioxidants that in turn help with tissue repair and increase your immunity.

The last four tests are infectious disease related. Epstein Barr Virus (EBV) is better known as mononucleosis. It is human herpesvirus 4, the most common human virus in the world. You do not have to have had mono to have EBV in your system. This one virus alone can reek havoc on your entire immune system, causing your thyroid to falter and ultimately causing your autoimmunity or inflammation. (It can be the cause of many autoimmune diseases. For this reason alone, I recommend testing for it). Herpes simplex 1 (HSV-1) causes oral herpes. Herpes simplex 2 (HSV-2) causes genital herpes. Once you've contracted EBV and/or HSV1/HSV2, you will always have it. This are viruses. They lay dormant in your body, causing your immune system to weaken and hence causing you problems.

Once you get your blood results back, pay attention to the "normal" range for each test. It is very possible your results come back "normal" but are on the very low or high end of the range. For example, my TSH (once I was treated) came back at 2.85. Which is in normal range, but my doctor wanted it at 1.0. Based on this, we adjusted mediation accordingly. Make sure you ask questions. Point out where your results are borderline and ask if these results could mean there is an underlying issue. Remember, you do not need to have an abnormal TSH result to have TPO and/or Thyroglobulin antibodies. The presence of these antibodies indicate there is an inflammation (autoimmunity) issue. Further, there is a direct correlation between autoimmunity (thyroid antibodies) and the presence of EBV. Testing positive for either of these and/or HSV1/HSV2, indicates inflammation in your body. The best and quickest way to feeling better is to address and treat this inflammation.

Further, always keep your lab results for your records. I personally have a large folder with all the paperwork, and a spreadsheet with dates, results and test ranges. This will help you see the "trends" in your blood work. For instance, my results indicate that during the winter months my TSH goes up and my vitamin D goes down. So, my doctor and I know to increase my thyroid medication and vitamin D during the winter months.

As you and your doctor are going through your results and ultimately coming up with a diagnosis and treatment plan, keep in mind the supplements and medication I list in this guide. Ask about the specific brands and if your doctor doesn't carry them, ask if they can order them for you and/or you can always buy some of them online.

INFLAMMATION

If you have Hashimoto's Thyroiditis, you have inflammation. If you have EBV and/or Herpes (active or non-active), you have inflammation. There is a direct correlation between Hashimoto's Thyroiditis and viral infections such as EBV and Herpes. If you tested negative for EBV and/or Herpes, my guess is you have another virus living silently in your body causing inflammation (measles, mumps, rubella, enteroviruses and parvoviruses have been linked to trigger Hashimoto's). Inflammation is the body's response to infections and damaged tissue. When you have a visible cut on the outside of your body, you can see the body's immune response to healing that cut. What makes inflammation on the inside of our body so hard to understand and notice, is that we can't see it. We don't know it's happening until we feel sick. Our immune system is an amazingly powerful response to this damage and foreign invaders inside our bodies. It's constantly working to defend us from harm. However, if the inflammation inside our bodies isn't addressed, our immune system becomes weak. When this happens, we end up with what the medical community calls Autoimmune Diseases like Hashimoto's, Graves', Rheumatoid Arthritis, Crohn's Disease, etc.

The quickest way to feeling better is by reducing this inflammation. I strongly recommend reading Anthony William's, *Medical Medium-Thyroid Healing*. Or any other book by Anthony William. Have you heard of the celery juice movement? Yep, that's him. He's a genius. Well worth the money and insight into inflammation in our bodies, how to reduce it and ultimately rid ourselves of it.

Make no mistake about it. The process of reducing inflammation in the body can take time. It does not happen overnight. The quickest response I had was by going on a gluten free diet. It wasn't easy. I loved pizza, beer and mac n' cheese. I absolutely hated it at first, but I told myself I'd give it six months before giving up. When I first had my TPO antibodies (IU/mL) tested they were 953. After going gluten free, they were 270. That's incredible! Not only did the blood work give me the proof that the inflammation was reducing, I FELT it! I had more energy, the headaches were gone and my stomach didn't hurt (irregularity fixed). But even with TPO antibodies at 270, I knew I had more inflammation to get rid of. My next step was going dairy free. Which was just absurd to me because I love cheese, but I wanted to find out what was fueling the inflammation. And what would you know, my TPO antibodies were undetected and within normal range six months later. This was crazy and fantastic all at the same time. I knew my gut was on the right path to healing and my inflammation was too. Sure, it took awhile to get used to the new diet and way of life, but if it meant a healthier version of me, I was in.

This process took the better part of a year, and could take even longer for some, so don't give up on it. Keep in mind you can always start small and work up to eliminating as many "toxins" as you can. An anti-inflammatory diet consists of fruits and vegetables, and avoids processed foods and meats. The internet is a great tool, with so much information out there - you choose what's best for you. So, try a change in your diet, go back to your doctor six months later and get your TPO antibodies checked. You'll have the proof.

Now, you don't want to hear this, but along with diet and reducing inflammation, comes exercise. You don't have to go overboard with it, just a good 20-40 minutes, 3-4 times a week. I promise you it's not that bad. Personally, I like taking walks because it's easier on my body. Find something that works for you. Go with a friend, or use it as your personal free time. Just commit to doing it. I also suggest finding time for relaxation. Both exercise and relaxation techniques aid in the reduction of inflammation. We live in such a fast paced environment, we could all use some downtime. Try meditation, a massage, or simply a hot bath a few times a week. Your body and mind will thank you for it.

SUPPLEMENTS AND MEDICATION

The following is a list of supplements that have worked wonders for me. With disciplined administration for the last 1-3 years, along with diet, exercise and relaxation - I feel amazing! Some of these can be purchased online, but some can only be purchased via your doctor. Again, it is very important that you and your doctor work together on your treatment plan. This guide is not meant as a substitution for your doctor, it is simply a guide to help point you in the right direction. It is to help you ask the right questions, get you to a quick diagnosis and a healthier you, all while saving you money and time along your healing journey.

SAM-e by Xymogen
Homocysteine Supreme by Designs for Health
ProbioMax Daily DF by Xymogen
L-Lysine by Designs for Health
XymoZyme by Xymogen
ActivNutrients by Xymogen
D3 5000 by Xymogen
Ester-C & Flavonoids by Pure Encapsulations
Turmeric Curcumin with Bioperine 1500mg by Bio Schwartz
Estro Block Pro Formula

SAMe is by far my favorite supplement, for so many reasons. S-Adenosyl methionine is a naturally occurring chemical found in the body (mainly produced and consumed in the liver) and its purpose is to regulate key functions in our cells. Its often referred to as the methyl donor. Lower levels of SAMe in the body doesn't allow for proper methyl group transfers to take place and can lead to liver disease and depression. If you have Hashimoto's, you have inflammation. Inflammation in the body causes the liver to be sluggish. Supplementing with additional SAMe helps the body regulate the necessary chemical reactions to feel at our best.

Homocysteine Supreme is basically a high dose of B vitamins in their methylated and phosphorylated forms (superior forms for metabolism). Healthy homocysteine levels are needed for a healthy immune system, detoxification, cardiovascular health, and brain health. If your homocysteine levels are not ideal, your red blood cells are abnormally larger than most. When they are too large, they don't function properly. This can lead to iron deficiency or anaemia, a lack of energy, extreme tiredness, muscle weakness and/or depression.

ProbioMax Daily DF is the best probiotic I've tried. Probiotics are the good bacteria and yeasts our digestive systems need. They help balance out the good and bad bacteria in the gut and keep it healthy. This, in turn, helps the body properly digest food and absorb vitamins and minerals.

L-Lysine is an essential amino acid. It is used in the body to synthesize proteins. It is used to help lower viral loads in the body. Many use it to reduce the occurrence of cold sores or an HSV-1 outbreak.

XymoZyme is a combination of essential digestive enzymes. In order to properly absorb all the nutrients we put into our bodies, we need these digestive enzymes. They help break down molecules into smaller, more easily absorbed substances.

ActivNutrients is a multivitamin and mineral supplement. It contains all the essential vitamins and minerals our bodies need on a daily basis. Further, they are formulated and combined for optimal absorption.

D3 5000 is a vitamin D supplement that's 5000 IUs of cholecalciferol per capsule. Those with Hashimoto's have been found to have lower levels of vitamin D. This form of vitamin D, cholecalciferol, is the most efficient at raising blood levels of the vitamin. Proper levels of vitamin D are essential to combat fatigue, muscle weakness, depression, anxiety and bone loss/weakness. Vitamin D levels should be tested and monitored routinely by your doctor. Too much vitamin D can be toxic. Most cases of toxicity have been reported in those taking 20,000 IUs or more per day.

Ester-C and flavonoids is a blend of vitamin C and flavonoids that provides enhanced vitamin C support. With Hashimoto's, our immune system can use all the help we can give it. Vitamin

C is essential for a healthy immune system.

Turmeric Curcumin with Bioperine is a supplement that has powerful anti-inflammatory benefits and is a great antioxidant. The Bioperine helps the body absorb the curcumin. This supplement is so beneficial to reducing inflammation and protecting the body from free radicals and oxidative damage.

Estro Block Pro helps the liver clear toxic estrogens and aids in the production of healthy estrogens. In today's environment, the overuse of plastics, pesticides, preservatives, processed foods and pollution, alters our bodies into treating these substances like estrogens. Too much xenoestrogen buildup is toxic and can cause hormonal imbalances, a sluggish liver and the retention of fat cells. Both men and women can benefit from removing these toxic estrogens.

If you have low ferritin, and ONLY if prescribed by a doctor, I recommend **Ferrochel** by Designs for Health. Note: Too much iron can be toxic, do not take if you don't know your ferritin level and are not being monitored by a doctor. If you are prescribed Ferrochel, always take it with Ester-C and never take it within 4 hours of your thyroid medication (if you take one).

If you have a high TSH level, you'll need a thyroid medication. I have tried the various Levothyroxine medications out there and can tell you that the natural thyroid medications work much better. I suggest **Armour Thyroid** or a **natural desiccated thyroid**. The dosage you will need will be determined by your doctor and for this you will need a prescription.

I also highly recommend IV therapy. If this is within your budget, find a place near you that has the **Myers Cocktail** nutritional IVs. This can get expensive but the nutrients (Calcium, magnesium, B-Vitamins and Vitamin C) are absorbed much better via IV than orally. Continue to take supplements orally when receiving these IVs. These take roughly 45 minutes to administer and cost approximately $150-$250 per IV.

If you've read one of Anthony William's books, you'll also enjoy the added benefits of a more natural way to heal your body. Things like wild blueberries, celery juice, aloe water and lemon water are part of my daily routine. I also take pure **Hawaiian Spirulina** by Nutrex Hawaii. Spirulina helps remove toxic heavy metals from our body and it is also a powerful antioxidant and anti-inflammatory supplement.

To help speed up healing a leaky gut, I take 3oz of organic **Bone Broth** 2/day. I also take **L-Glutamine** by Xymogen daily.

CONCLUSION

Implementing all of this information at once would be overwhelming. This is a lot of research, data and results that took years to compile. Take it slow. Start with finding the right doctor and getting blood results. Once you and you're doctor are ready, start implementing new supplements and/or medications gradually. You'll want to see and feel how your body is reacting to a specific change and know it is working for you. If you implement everything all at once and you don't like the way you feel, how will you know which supplement or medication caused that reaction?

Remember, it takes time to heal and reduce inflammation. Implementing a new way of life isn't easy. Try to surround yourself with people that motivate and care about you. You are not alone. You can follow me on Instagram at hashimotosurvialguide and/or on Twitter at hashimotosurvi1. Further, there are plenty of other people out there that can provide support and information. I believe you can do it! Best of luck and cheers to a healthier you!!